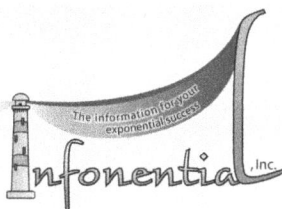

SOP Workshop

Workshop in a Book on Standard Operating Procedures for Biotechnology, Health Science, and Other Industries

Paul Sanghera, Ph.D.

SOP Workshop: Workshop in a Book on Standard Operating Procedures for Biotechnology, Health Science, and Other Industries

Published by
Infonential, Inc.
A California Corporation.
http://www.infonentialinc.com
email: info@infonentialinc.com

ISBN-10: 0-9791797-8-5
ISBN-13: 978-0-9791797-8-5

This publication is designed to provide accurate and authoritative information on the covered subject matter. It can be used by students and professionals in biotechnology, health sciences, and other industries that use standard operating procedures. However, it is sold with the understanding that the publisher is not engaged in offering technical, legal, or other professional service. If such assistance is required, the service of a competent professional should be sought.

To
The students and professionals in
The fields of
Biotechnology and health sciences

Table of Contents

The Workshop in a Book Series

The purpose of a *workshop in a book* is to present the required information on a subject within a well defined scope by focusing on the customer needs.

The lack of information is the problem of the past ages. The problem of the current age, the information age, is that we have too much information and too little time to absorb it. We are being bombarded with all kinds of needed and (mostly) un-needed information from all sides. This situation has created the need for information products that contain well defined, precise, to the point, quick, and "just what the customer needs" information. The *workshop in a Book Series* is a response to this market need. In other words, a *workshop in a book* is based on the philosophy that in this fast paced information age, nobody has the time to prowl through web pages or struggle with a 700 pages long book to find just that little piece of needed information.

Bottom line: A *workshop in a book* offers maximum learning in minimum time. No fluff, just the nuggets of the needed information presented in an easy to understand format.

About the Author

Dr. Paul Sanghera, an educator, scientist, technologist, and an entrepreneur, has a diverse background in all the fields on which biotechnology and health sciences are based including physics, chemistry, biology, computer science, and math. He holds a Master degree in Computer Science from Cornell University, a Ph.D. in Physics from Carleton University, and a B.Sc. with triple major: physics, chemistry, and math. He has taught science and technology courses all across the world including San Jose State University and Brooks College. Dr. Sanghera has been involved in educational programs and research projects in biotechnology. He has authored and co-authored more than 100 research papers published in well reputed European and American research journals.

As a technology manager, Dr. Sanghera has been at the ground floor of several technology startups. His responsibilities included process development and quality assurance at companies such as Netscape and MP3. He is the author of several best selling books in the fields of science, technology, and project management. He lives in Silicon Valley, California, where he currently serves as Adjunct Professor at California Institute of Nanotechnology.

x

About This Book

Format: lecture notes which are:

- ❖ self-contained
- ❖ presented in a logical and easy-to-follow sequence
- ❖ Comprehensive and complete within the scope of this book

Who can benefit from this workshop?

- ❖ Professionals in biotechnology, healthcare, and other industries that use SOPs
- ❖ Students of biotechnology and health sciences
- ❖ Managers and executives for a quick review of how to implement SOP system within their organizations

Topics:

- ❖ Introduction to SOPs
- ❖ Effective SOPs
- ❖ Producing Effective SOPs
- ❖ Living with Approved SOPs
- ❖ Process Based Approach to SOPs
- ❖ Solutions to Self Test Exercises
- ❖ Glossary

Why Should You Care?

Failure to follow one's own procedures is the single most-cited violation of the GMP regulations.

1

Introduction to SOPs

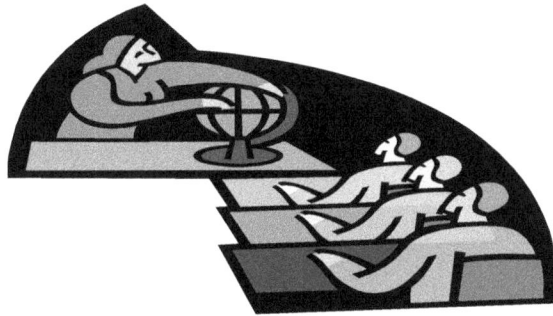

1. SOP: Definition

2. Why SOPs

3. SOPs in Biotechnology and Health Industry

4. Purpose and advantages of SOPs

5. Implementing SOPs

6. A Simple Example

7. Summary and Conclusions

8. Self Test Exercises

Introduction to SOPs

What is SOP?

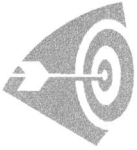

- **Standard Operating Procedure (SOP)**: A document that contains a set of instructions with the power of directives to perform a procedure or operation effectively.

- "…detailed, written instructions to achieve uniformity of the performance of a specific function."

  International Conference on Harmonisation (ICH)

- "…written procedures that accurately describe and detail essential job tasks." *FDA*

Used in several fields such as healthcare, education, IT industry, and military.

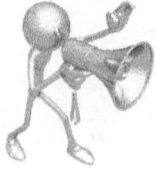

A popular Misconception: SOPs are standardized across a given industry.

This is of course false. SOPs for a given procedure are written, modified, and approved at an organizational level.

In nutshell:

Procedures and processes under which we operate are standardized so that:

1. A given procedure is performed the same way each time.

2. A given procedure is performed the same way by each person.

These two points bring uniformity and consistency to procedures and operations.

Mantra behind SOPs:

Write down what you are going to do; do what is written down.

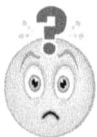

Can two organizations have different SOPs for the same procedure/ operation?

A: Yes, and they often do.

Introduction to SOPs

Why SOP?

SOPs cover those tasks, processes, operations, or features that lend themselves to standardized procedure without loss of effectiveness.

General Advantages

- Effective SOPs can act as catalysts to improve the results of an operation and organization's overall performance.

- SOPs are the most fundamental component of current Good Manufacturing Practices (cGMP).

- SOP compliance improves quality control. In fact, SOPs are essential components of good quality assurance (QA) and quality control (QC) systems.

- SOPs are means to achieve uniformity in the performance of a specific function.

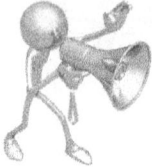

A good quality assurance (QA) system and a good quality control (QC) system is based on SOPs.

In nutshell

The purpose of an SOP is to ensure that essential job tasks are performed consistently, correctly, and in conformance with internally approved procedures which include regulatory requirements.

⬇

The correct and consistent performance of essential job tasks addresses both quality as well as regulatory requirements.

In some fields and situations, SOPs are legally required

SOP: Legal Requirement

Regulations, for example by the FDA in the U.S., require SOPs.

The bottom lines are:

- You shall write down how you will perform your procedures.
- You shall get your procedures approved.
- You shall follow the approved written procedures.
- When a part of the approved written procedure is not followed, you shall open a deviation and investigate it.

Based on 21CFR211.100

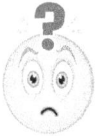

What is CFR?

> **A:** Code of Federal Regulations.

SOPs in Biotechnology and Health Industry

- SOPs are necessary for a clinical research for performing clinical research operations in order to maximize safety and optimize efficiency and effectiveness.
- All sites involved in clinical studies must have SOPs to ensure compliance with the current regulations.
- One of the motivations is to protect the safety and welfare of study subjects.
- SOPs are an integral part of the clinical trials at all levels including investigative sites, sponsors, and institutional review boards (IRB). For example:

  > The ICH GCP (good clinical practice) Step 5 Guideline (Section 3.2.2) suggests that an Institutional Review Board (IRB) have its own SOPs or written standard procedures.

Introduction to SOPs

The presence of properly written, maintained, and followed SOPs is essential when inspections take place.

Most frequent reported deficiencies during inspections are the lack of written SOPs, the failure to adhere to them, or boyh. The risk of GCP non-compliance is high at organizations with the following situations:

- A poor availability of SOPs specific to clinical research
- SOPs are available but their persumpted users who need to follow them are either not aware of them or don't follow them. → Need for training.

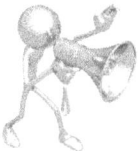

SOPs can play important role in fulfilling the ICH, FDA and other regulatory requirements.

Investing in Ensuring

Writing and Adhering to Good SOPs Ensure or Help to Ensure the Following:

- The site has uniform and consistent processes that meet the regulatory and good clinical practice (GCP) standards.

- The site has a proper control over its operations, procedures, and processes.

- The employees are familiar with the processes.

- The processes are reviewed and updated on a regular basis as needed or required.

- The audits by sponsors, FDA, or other regulatory agencies do not result in detrimental findings and citations.

- The site has some legal protection.

More on Advantages of SOPs

- A clinical research organization that writes, maintains, and follows good SOPs has distinct advantage over those that do not.

- The SOP system prompts an organization to interpret and apply GCP guidelines to its operations, which is critical.

- SOPs help ensure accountability, compliance, and consistency from personnel at all levels of an organization.

- Clinical research organizations without SOPs run a high risk of GCP non-compliance and poor productivity.

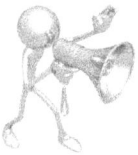

On these few pages we have discussed SOPs in context of clinical organizations, but writing and using SOPs is not limited to just this type of organizations.

Critical Steps in Implementing SOPs

1. Produce SOPs

2. Review SOPs

3. Approve SOPs

4. Use SOPs

5. Monitoring and control SOPs, which include managing:

   o implementations

   o modifications

Implementing SOPs: Big Picture

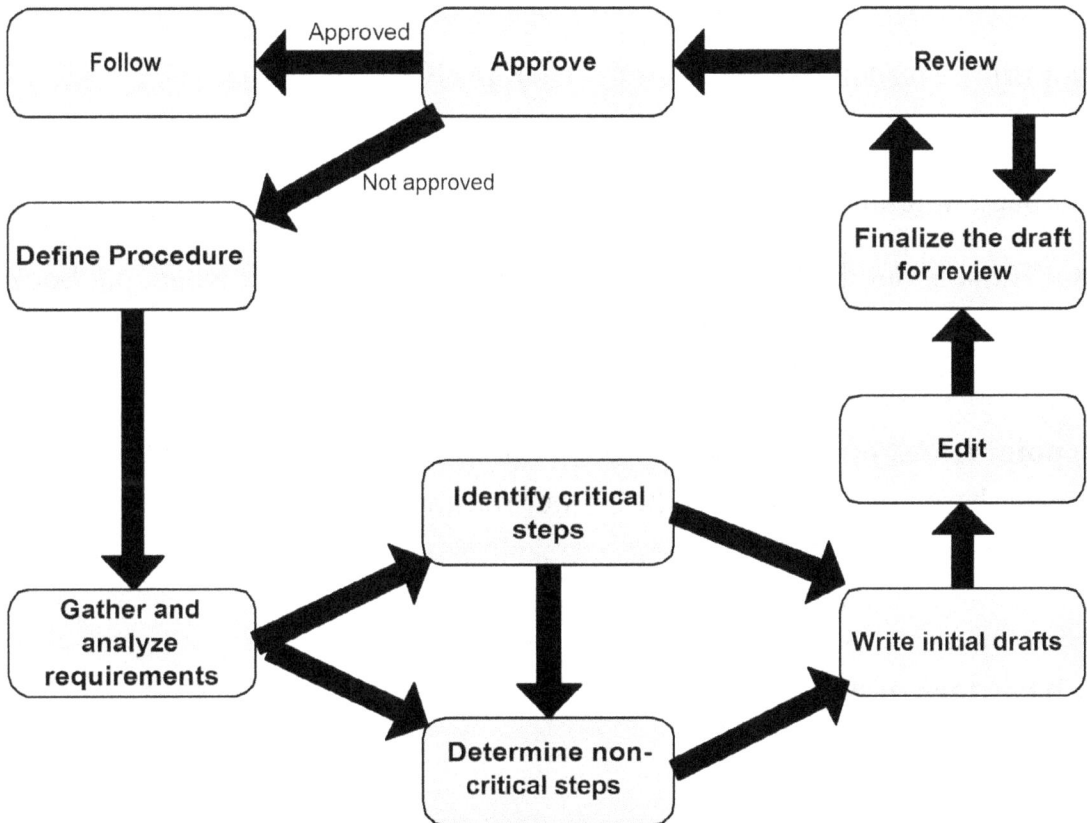

```
┌──────────┐  Approved   ┌──────────┐         ┌──────────┐
│  Follow  │◄────────────│ Approve  │◄────────│  Review  │
└──────────┘             └──────────┘         └──────────┘
                           │    ▲                ▲   │
                    Not approved                 │   ▼
┌─────────────────┐       ▼              ┌──────────────────┐
│ Define Procedure│◄──                   │ Finalize the draft│
└─────────────────┘                      │    for review     │
      │                                  └──────────────────┘
      ▼                                           ▲
┌─────────────────┐    ┌─────────────┐     ┌──────────┐
│  Gather and     │    │Identify      │     │   Edit   │
│  analyze        │───►│critical steps│     └──────────┘
│  requirements   │──  └─────────────┘            ▲
└─────────────────┘  ─  │        ────►  ┌────────────────────┐
                   ─    ▼          │    │ Write initial drafts│
                    ──►┌─────────────┐──►└────────────────────┘
                       │Determine non-│
                       │critical steps│
                       └─────────────┘
```

Big picture: Typical flow among various steps involved in implementing an SOP

So, You Say You Have Never Seen an SOP

If you think you have never seen or used an SOP, think again:

- Think about the basic general definition of an SOP presented in the beginning of this module.

- Think about the last time you followed a recipe in the kitchen, put book shelf together by reading the manual that came with the book shelf components in a box, and so on.

The point is: All of us perform different kinds of operations, procedures, and processes based on instructions during our routine life

⇓

The basic idea of an SOP should not be a foreign concept to us.

SOP: A Ridiculously Simple Example

Procedure:

You have bought uncooked pizza and you intend to put some toppings on it and cook it in the oven in your kitchen. The instructions on the pizza wrap suggest preheating the oven to 425° C and cook for 18 minutes. You want to cook your pizza.

First, the instructions on the pizza wrap can be considered an SOP in itself.

Second, you can write your own SOP for this operation.

Example:

SOP 1.1: Cooking Pizza

1. Turn the oven on and set the temperature to 425°C. The pre-heating starts.

2. Put the toppings on the pizza.

3. When the oven has been pre-heated to 425°C, it will beep.

4. Upon the beep, put the pizza into the oven.

5. Set the timer to 18 minutes.

6. When the timer beeps, peep at the pizza in the oven. If it has been cooked to your liking, turn the oven off, take the pizza out, and you are done; else go to step 7.

7. Set the timer for 2 minutes.

8. Go back to step 6.

Introduction to SOPs

Summary and Conclusions

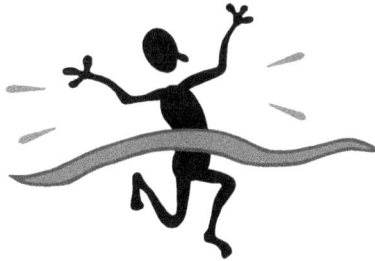

- A standard operating procedure (SOP) is a document that contains accurate and detailed instructions to perform a process, procedure, or operation.

- SOPs are the most fundamental component of the current Good Manufacturing Practices (cGMPs).

- SOPs re required in the life sciences industry.

- SOPs are not industry wide standards; they are written, used, and managed within an organization.

- Good quality assurance (QA) and Quality Control (QC) systems are based on SOPs.

- The main purpose of an SOP is to ensure that essential job tasks are performed consistently, accurately, and in conformance with the approved procedures within the organization.

- Good SOPs:
    - ✓ help improve performance and effectiveness of operations
    - ✓ provide proper control over operations
    - ✓ provide legal protection

Introduction to SOPs

Self Test Exercises

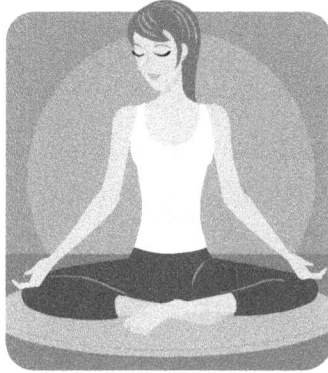

1 What is an SOP?

2 **True or False**: SOPs in clinical industry are documents standardized for the whole industry that describe how to perform certain operations.

3 **True or False**: SOPs are only used in biotechnology and health industry.

4 **True or False**: SOPs are only used to meet regulatory requirements.

5 Each SOP has a start point of an operation and the finish point. In SOP 1.1 for cooking pizza presented in module 1, identify the start point and the finish point.

6 SOPs often have assumptions, for example, they may assume that there is something that the user already knows and does not need to be written down. Identify at least one assumption in SOP 1.1 for cooking pizza.

7 An SOP may have a flexibility built into it. Identify at least one flexibility built into SOP 1.1 for cooking pizza.

2

Effective SOPs

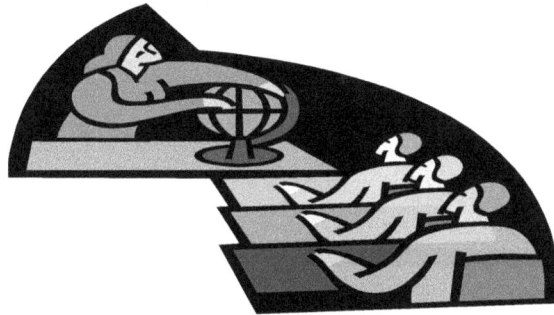

1. Effective SOP: Definition

2. Producing Effective SOPs: Challenges

3. Components of an Effective SOP System

4. Document Management System

5. Managing Changes to SOPs

What is an Effective SOP?

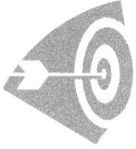

Effective SOP. An SOP that is capable of producing the intended results.

An effective SOP tends to have the following characteristics:

- **Complete**. Contains all the information needed to perform the procedure.
- **Clear and concise.** Provides to-the-point information in short and easy to understand sentences.
- **Coherent**. Logical flow in two ways:
    - There is a logical flow throughout the content of the SOP.
    - The steps necessary to complete procedure are presented in the sequence in which they will be executed.
- **Objective**. Based on facts and not opinions or likes and dislikes.

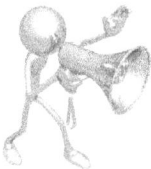

An effective SOP avoids long and wordy sentences. It communicates the whole information in the fewest possible words, sentences, and steps/paragraphs. It is easy to follow.

Challenges to Produce Effective SOPs

- You need to integrate many skills together such as expertise in the subject matter and good writing skills: not everyone or every expert is a good writer.

- The effective SOP has to work for all users with varying backgrounds.

- It may be time consuming to write an effective SOP. You need to make a good judgment call when it's good enough.

- You need to strike a balance or a tradeoff between cost and benefit: again a judgment call.

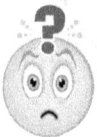

How do you define an effective SOP?

Effective SOPs

Defining an Effective SOP

Effective SOPs don't just appear; they need to be defined for a given procedure, designed/planned, and produced.

Steps for defining effective SOPs include the following:

- Define the effective procedure for which the SOP will be written, for example, identify requirements of the procedure.

- Determine how quality of the written procedure will be measured.

- Define success:
    - What are the factors or results that will determine the success of the procedure to be written in the SOP?
    - What are the factors or results that will determine the success of the SOP?

- Cost benefit analysis: how much will it cost to produce and implement effective SOPs and how does the cost compare to its benefits?

An effective SOP is a "good SOP" from the user's perspective.

Good SOP: From a User's Perspective

- Easy to follow
- Tells what's critical to execute or control
- Warns about the safety issues
- Other than the built-in flexibility, there is no vagueness: each user can follow it and perform the procedure in the same way.
- Minimizes the probability for errors and mixups.
- Uses good technical writing tools and techniques such as visuals.
- Short and a good read.

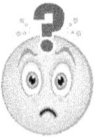

What does it take to put an effective SOP system in place?

Components of an Effective SOP System

- **Templates**. Wherever/whenever possible, design and use templates to write SOPs. It will help save time and implement uniformity and consistency.

- **Readers**. A given SOP should have well defined readers (users) and should be written primarily for them.

- **Structure**. Use structural elements such as sections, numbered steps, warnings, forms, and tables. This will help make the SOP easy to follow.

- **Expertise**. SOP writers and reviewers will need certain expertise such as the subject matter expertise. If a writer or a reviewer does not have a needed expertise, the needed expert judgment from experts can be used.

- **Document management system.** Such a system is needed to manage development of SOPs, maintain their integrity, and control changes to them.

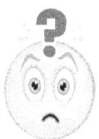

What is a document management system and why do you need it?

Document Management System

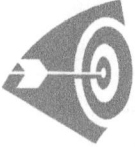

Document management system (DMS). A computerized system that consists of computers and software programs running on them to manage documents.

Managing a document may include:
- ✓ Developing the document.
- ✓ Accepting feedback/reviews
- ✓ Controlling changes to the document
- ✓ Making the document obsolete when needed

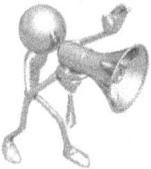

Even if you use paper-based SOPs, you can use the DMS to develop, maintain, and control them.

Why DMS?

Advantages:

- **Automation**. Automates development and management tasks ➔ saves time, increases efficiency, and enhances relaibility.

- **Tracability**. Ensures that you can always find the desired document with the right version.

- **Integrity.** Ensures that the information cannot be changed by unauthorized personnel.

- **Changes**. Can be used to ensure that:
  - A correct change history is maintained.
  - The changes are controlled properly.

- **Integration**. Can be easily integrated with othe rsystem and databases of the company for mutual benefits and to increase performance and efficiency.

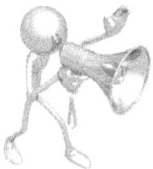

Change control includes accepting change proposals, approving/disapproving changes, and implementing the improved changes. Change control should be the responsibility of QA.

DMS in a Big Picture

If you join a start-up company it may not yet have a document management system in place, whereas an established company may already have a DMS either stand alone or as a part of another system such as the following:

> **Configuration management system (CMS).** A system that manages the following characteristics of a product:

- o identity
- o consistency
- o change control
- o status accounting
- o verification
- o auditing

Change control may be part of the configuration management system or it may also be a stand-alone system.

➤ **Change control system (CCS).** A collection of formal documented procedures that specify how certain entities such as project plans and scopes, and other documents will be:
  o controlled
  o changed
  o approved

The system may exist as an automated computer system that implements these procedures. There is obviously an overlap between configuration management system and change control system.

➤ **Content management system (CMS).** A computerized system used to create, store, edit, control, and retrieve (or publish) content in a consistent and automated fashion.

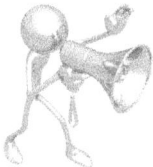

A good practice: Destroying a document should require the consent of at least two individuals.

Maintaining Change History

- **Linkage**. Change history should be part of (or properly linked to) an effective SOP.

- **Traceability**. Change history should be easily traceable, for example, answers to questions like the following must be readily available:

  - How was a given procedure performed at a specific time in the past?

  - How is this procedure performed now?

  - What are the changes, when were they made, and why?

- **Integrity**. You should make sure that a change in one SOP does not undermine the integrity of other SOPs. *Example*: An existing SOP refers to another SOP that was made obsolete in the past.

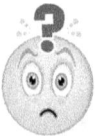

How do I know an SOP is an effective SOP?

Measuring SOP Effectiveness

Measuring the effectiveness of an SOP is a two step process:

1. **Collect the data on the SOP usage**:

   - **Interviews**. Interview the SOP users to find out what troubles they had with its usage and what features were helpful.

   - **Deviations**. How many deviations have happened and how often each deviation has been happening.

   - **Changes**. How many times the SOP has been revised.

   - **Training**. How much training and re-training was needed for the SOP users?

2. **Analyze this data to determine and measure:**

   - The strong points about the SOP

   - The weak points about the SOP

   - The success factors and metrics

Maintaining the Effectiveness of SOPs

Keeping your SOP effective involves accepting the following facts and dealing with them head-on:

- **Errors.** Errors do happen. Keep your SOP as error-proof as possible by doing the following:

  o Identify the errors.

  o Eliminate the errors as they are identified and make necessary repair.

  o Learn from the errors as they occur to do better in the future.

- **Mixups.** Watch out for the possibility of mixups and guard your SOP against them.

- **Following SOPs.** No SOP will be effective until it is properly followed.

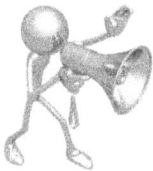

1. Mix-ups are the most common cause for the occurrence of patient adverse events in hospitals.

2. Failure to follow SOPs, that is, to follow procedures exactly as written, is the most common FDA citation in U.S.A.

Effective SOPs

Some Common Grievances about SOPs

Producing and maintaining an effective SOP may include addressing one or more of the following common grievances about SOPs:

- **Time consuming**. It takes too long to write and review SOPs.

- **Role problem**. Each reviewer rewrites an SOP to his/her own liking.

- **Clarity**. SOPs make no sense.

- **Errors**. SOPs have factual errors.

- **References**. SOPs lack references or refer to documents that are not available or have been made obsolete.

- **Compliance**. For example, SOPs do not comply with cGMP.

- **Erroneously Inclusive**. SOPs have sweeping terms in them such as "applied to everybody", whereas in practice they are applied to only certain departments or groups.

Summary and Conclusions

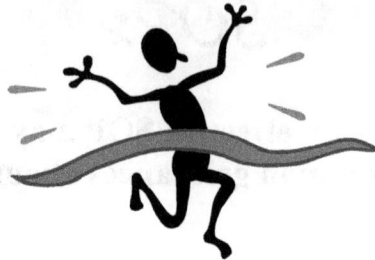

- An Effective SOP is an SOP that is capable of producing the intended results.

- An Effective SOP is complete, concise, coherent, objective, and easy to follow.

- An effective SOP works well for all users.

- A document management system facilitates developing and managing effective SOPs.

- It's important to manage the change history and make it part of the SOP.

- No SOP can be effective if it's not followed properly. Failure to follow SOPs, that is, to follow procedures exactly as written, is the most common FDA citation in the U.S.A.

- Mixups are the most common cause for the occurrence of patient adverse events in hospitals. An effective SOP minimizes the possibility of mixups.

Effective SOPs

Self Test Exercises

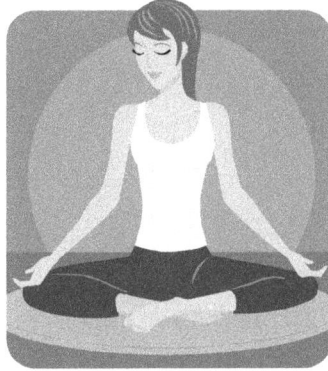

1 You have just made an SOP obsolete. There are three existing SOPs that refer to this SOP. What will you do to maintain the effectiveness of those SOPs?

2 Most employees have deviated step 5 of your SOP most of the time. What is the most likely problem? Suggest a solution.

3 One employee has deviated step 5 of your SOP most of the times. Other employees are using this SOP as well, and they are not deviating. What is the most likely problem? Suggest a solution.

4 Changes in SOPs must be controlled by:

A. Authors of the SOPs

B. QA

C. CEO of the company

D. Manager of the users

Effective SOPs

3

Producing Effective SOPs

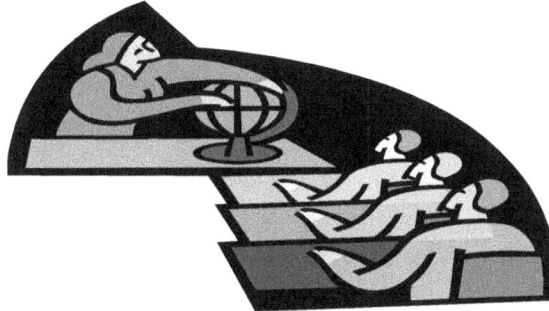

1. *Definition*

2. *Process of Writing an SOP*

3. *Anatomy of an SOP*

4. *Good Technical Writing*

5. *Common Pitfalls*

6. *Reviewing SOPs*

7. *Quality Cycle*

Producing an Effective SOP: Big Picture

Producing an effective SOP includes:

- Writing SOP
- Reviewing SOP
- Approving SOP

After all these efforts, you follow it!

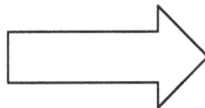

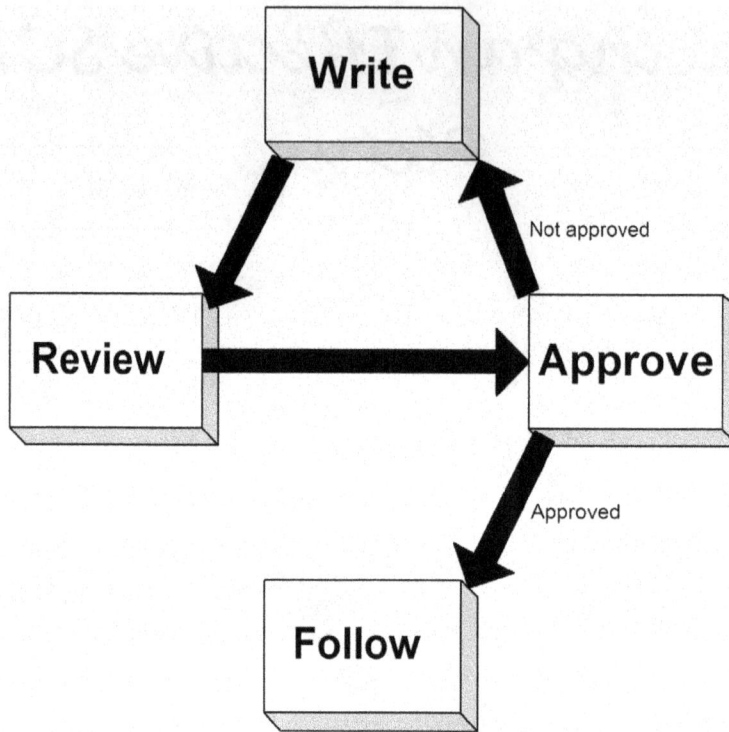

Typical flow among writing, reviewing, approving, and following SOPs

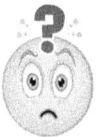

What is the process of writing an SOP?

Process of Writing an SOP

An SOP is written for a procedure:

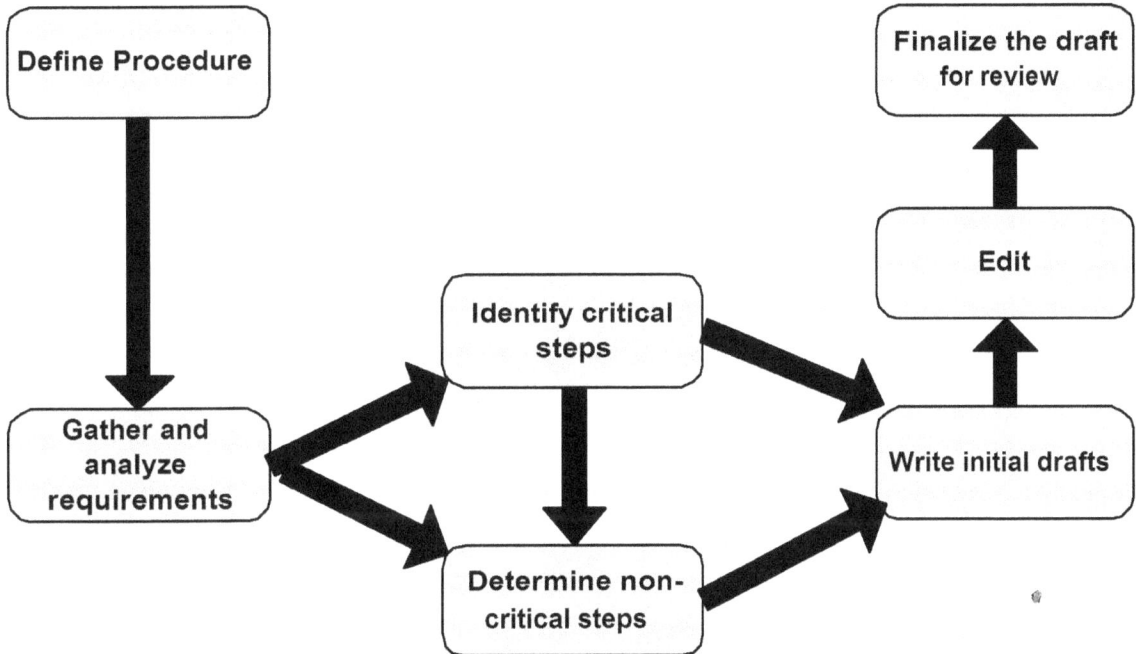

Typical flow among various steps involved in writing an SOP

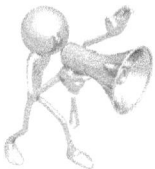

In a project based organization, an SOP can be written as a project or as a part of a project. In project management, a process has an input, and you use some tools and techniques to produce output from the input.

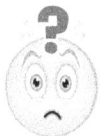

What are the input, tools and techniques, and output of the process of writing an SOP?

Process of Writing an SOP: Elements

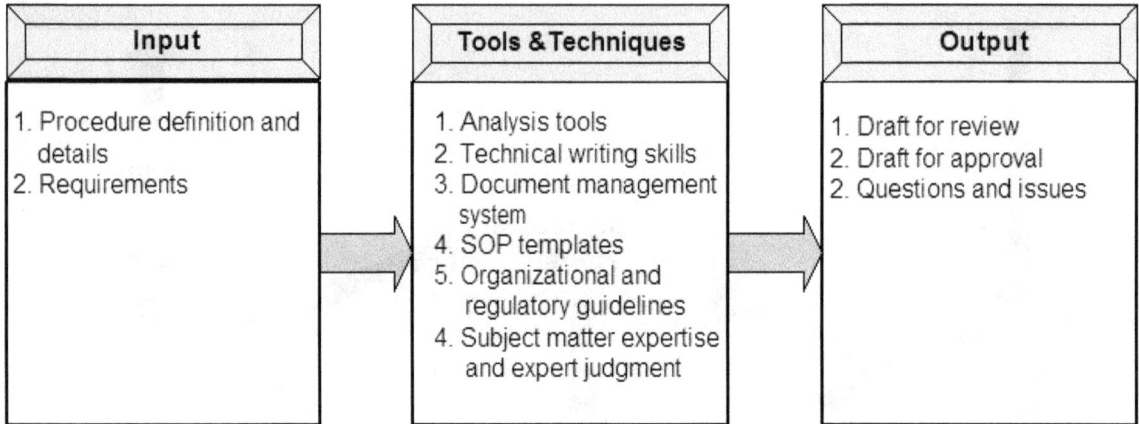

Input	Tools & Techniques	Output
1. Procedure definition and details 2. Requirements	1. Analysis tools 2. Technical writing skills 3. Document management system 4. SOP templates 5. Organizational and regulatory guidelines 4. Subject matter expertise and expert judgment	1. Draft for review 2. Draft for approval 2. Questions and issues

The write SOP process

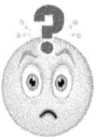

OK, I understand the process, but how do you execute it?

Producing Effective SOPs

Writing an SOP: Some Steps

- Define the procedure about which the SOP is to be written.
- Gather and analyze requirements:
    - Gather procedure related requirements.
    - Find out compliance requirements.
    - Find out roles and responsibilities such as the readers of the SOP, the reviewers, and the person who will approve it.
    - Determine reader requirements.
    - Define success, for example, through a set of metrics.
- Determine the steps of the procedure:
    - Critical steps
    - Non-critical steps
    - Details: execution of steps, in between thew steps, and warnings etc.
- Arrange the steps in sequenc in which the procedure will be executed.
- Fill in the necessary details

Anatomy of an SOP

Some Common Sections/elements of an SOP:

- **SOP number**
- **Title**
- **Purpose.** Specify the purpose of the SOP and the procedure that is described in the SOP.
- **List of equipment or material used in the procedure**
- **Roles and responsibilities**
- **Scope**, for example, whom this SOP applies to
- **Procedure**. The steps and the details of the procedure to be performed
- **Summary**
- **Change History**

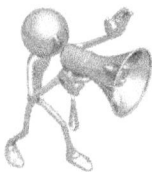

Either avoid using the sweeping terms in the scope such as "this SOP applies to all..." or use them with great caution. Be more specific in specifying the scope, for example, by stating what is included and what is excluded.

Producing Effective SOPs

Knowing the Readers

- Identify all the readers, for example:
    - Users such as research associates and lab technicians
    - QA
    - Your boss
    - FDA investigators
- Identify the primary and secondary users.
- Determine the following about the readers:
    - Level of expertise or understanding of the procedure
    - Technical experience and background
    - Language fluency
- Gather and analyze the user requirements.

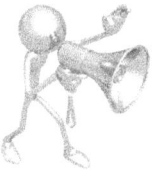

Write your SOP for the readers, primarily for the users.

Technical Writing Tools and Techniques

Use the following tools and techniques wherever appropriate in the SOP:

- Tables
- Graphs
- Illustrations and figures
- Lists
- Forms
- Flow charts
- Standard terminology
- Standardized format and templates
- Examples
- Background information

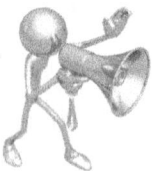

The whole purpose of using these tools is to facilitate comprehension, make the SOP easy to follow, and thereby minimize the probability of making mistakes and errors.

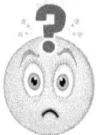

What defines a good form?

Defining a Good Form

Characteristics of an effectively designed form:

- The form design simple and clear
- Information asked in a logical sequence and aligned with the procedure
- Enough space provided to enter the information
- Field names chosen properly, and non-obvious field names explained
- Good design principles such as:
    - Clear and easy to follow
    - Error proof
    - Appropriate elements: radio buttons, check boxes, text input box

Characteristics of a Poorly designed form:

- Difficult to use
- Lacks adequate space to write in
- Does not follow the order of the steps in the SOP
- Does not match with SOP
- Disagrees with the SOP

Tips from Good Technical Writing

- **Apply Preacher's Axiom**: *"Tell the readers what you are going to tell them, then tell them, and then tell them what you have just told them."* All it means that the SOP and each of its sections contain:
  - A brief introductory description followed by
  - Complete description with details followed by
  - Conclusion that summarizes the main points that were covered
- **Use numbered list**. Give the instructions to perform a process in a numbered list that lists the steps to be executed in the order of execution.
- **Make it more direct,** for example, use active voice as opposed to passive voice:

  Active: QA *reviewed and approved* the document.

  Passive: The document *was reviewed and approved*.

- **Use the terms to draw attention to risks** such as caution, warning, and danger. Provide the risk information about a step before you ask the user to execute the step.
- **Leave out clichés.**
- **Be accurate.** Distinguish facts from opinions.

- **Use absolute words carefully.** Examples: all, never, maximize, minimize.

- **Use nonsexist language**.

Say it with a Style

- Write clear sentences
- Be concise
- Be accurate in wording
- Use the active voice
- Use the non-sexist language
- Avoid jargon/slang
- Refer to other existing controlled documents, and not to memos, emails etc.

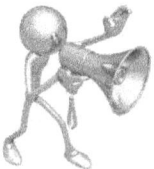

Make it easy to read
Make it easy to succeed

Slippery Words

Use the words like the following very carefully (or avoid them if you can):

- All, none
- Always, never
- Exactly
- Almost, about
- As appropriate
- But
- Equivalent
- If required

Common Pitfalls in Writing an SOP

- Assuming the wrong technical level of the users, e.g. too much technical expertise, and thereby using the technical jargon that the readers will not understand

- Using local jargon (e.g. lab slangs) that all users may not be aware of

- Assuming that all users (readers) know certain things about your company, lab, product, and QA/QC systems

- No logical flow and lots of hopping around

- Leaving out an important step assuming it's obvious

- Too much detail about trivial matters

- No examples, figures, or other aid for the users to follow the procedure properly

- Redundant instructions

- Lack of specificity where it is needed

- Poorly designed forms: not enough space provided to write in a field, don't match the procedure, and so on

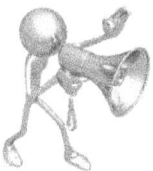

Road-test your SOP before making it law. Uncaught errors in SOPs can lead to fatal accidents and deaths. Example: a patient dies after receiving 20 mg of medication instead of 2.0 mg due to badly written and erroneously read prescription.

Common Errors in writing/reading SOPs

- Misinterpretations and misreading

- Executing steps in a wrong sequence

- Inventing new (your own) process during reading or writing

- Skipping a step

- Transcription error, that is, copying error

- Transposal error, for example, reading 37 for 73

- Calculation errors, for example, different users may use different significant figures in their calculations

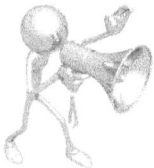

Once you know the errors that the readers will potentially make, you can take steps to make your SOP as much error proof as possible.

Essentials of Reviewing SOPs

- Who are the Reviewers?
- Checking for Accuracy
- Checking for Redundancy and gaps
- Checking for Quality
- Review it; do not re-write it

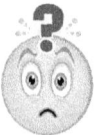

So, who are the reviewers?

The SOP Reviewers

Who are they?

Depending on the content of the SOP, there may be multiple reviewers of your SOP belonging to different departments such as:

- QA
- QC
- Development
- Lab management
- Manufacturing
- Training
- Facilities
- Purchasing

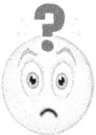

How does checking for accuracy work?

Checking for Accuracy

Checking for accuracy includes ensuring:

- All steps are there; clearly written.
- All steps are in the correct sequence.
- SOP is based on facts and not opinions.
- Wording is accurate.
- SOP complies with *cGMP*.

Review also includes checking for redundancy and gaps

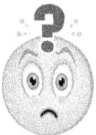

What do you mean by checking for redundancy and gaps?

Producing Effective SOPs

Checking for Redundancy and Gaps

- Check for unnecessary trivial details.
- Check for the repetition of the same set of instructions.
- Check the gap between the reader's technical level and what level is assumed in the SOP.
- Check if an essential step is skipped.

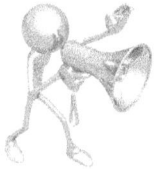

If there are too many unnecessary trivial details, the reader may focus on the wrong aspect. If the SOP is too long, the reader may shy away from reading it altogether.

Review also includes checking for quality

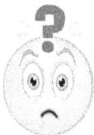

How do you check for quality?

Checking for Quality

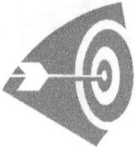

Quality of a product, SOP in this case, is the degree to which its characteristics meet the planned requirements and objectives.

Checking for quality:

- Check that the SOP meets all the cGMP requirements.
- Check that the SOP meets all the requirements set by the QA/QC department.
- Check for accuracy and readability.
- Check for general writing quality features.
- Be aware of the general rules of modern quality management.

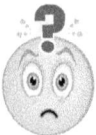

What are the rules of modern quality management?

Guiding Rules of Modern Quality Management

- **Putting the customer first**. The customers in this case are the readers, primarily the users.

- **Prevention over inspection**. The cost of preventing mistakes and errors is much less than the cost of correcting them after being revealed by inspection.

- **Management responsibility**. It's the responsibility of the management to provide resources needed for the success of any product or project.

- **Continuous improvement**. Follow the plan-do-check-act cycle for the quality improvement.

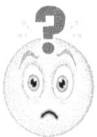

What is the plan-do-check-act cycle?

The Quality Cycle

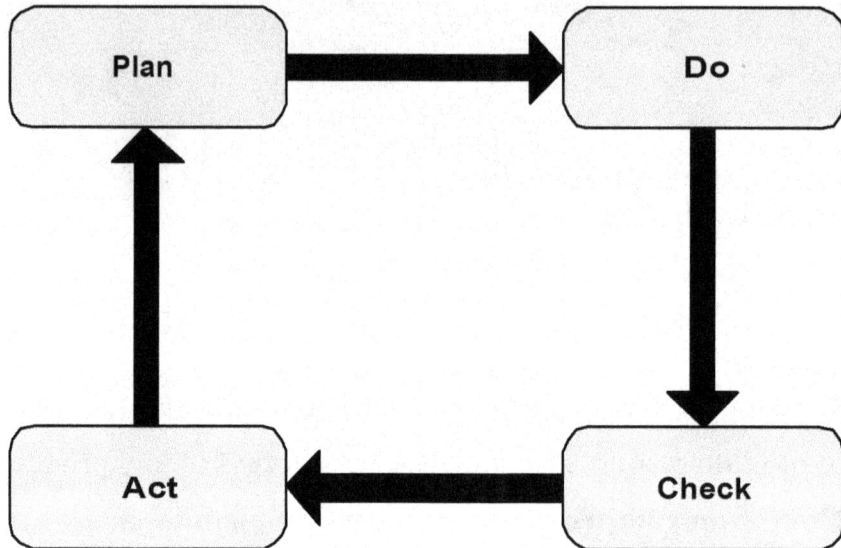

The Plan-Do-Check-Act cycle defined by
Schewhart and modified by Deming.

Applying to SOP writing, it means:

1. Plan the SOP

2. Write the SOP as planned

3. Check (review) the SOP

4. Implement the necessary changes

5. Modify the plan if needed, and so on...

Getting Reviews in a Timely Fashion

- Plan/schedule them, that is, tell the reviewers, an SOP is coming for a review.

- Notify the reviewers if the SOP draft for them is going to be delayed.

- Provide the document: Make it easily accessible.

- Follow up.

- Appreciate the reviewers.

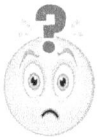

After the review, how is the SOP approved?

Approving SOPs

- Usually, the QA department within a company approves the SOP.

- You should check out what if any are the regulatory guidelines in your industry and in your company for getting the SOP approved.

- Your company may have approval requirements in addition to approval from the QA.

- Once approved, SOP must be followed just like law.

Summary and Conclusion

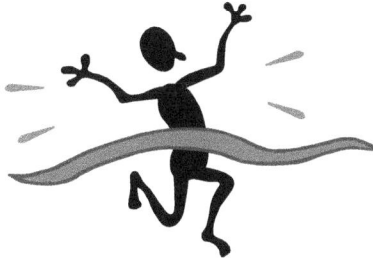

- Producing an SOP includes writing, reviewing, and approving the SOP.

- Procedure definition and requirements are some of the input items for the process of writing an SOP.

- Analysis tools, document management system, and technical writing skills are some of the tools and techniques that you use to produce SOP from the input.

- SOP should contain all the needed information and must not be too long.

- Having said that it should fulfill all the requirements, an SOP is basically written for its primary readers, the users.

- An SOP should have a structure and should be written by using the good technical writing practices.

- While writing, take steps to make your SOP error proof.

- Before sending your SOP for approval, get it reviewed by designated individuals and groups.

- Before the SOP is followed, it must be approved by the designated individuals within your company.

- After the SOP is approved, it must be followed like law.

Self Test Exercises

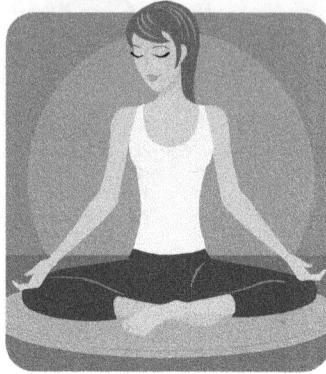

1 You see a signboard that reads the following:

Chemicals that are known to be dangerous to your health are used in this facility!

This warning is suffering from which pitfall?

2 What are the possible results of vague instructions for a procedure?

3 Read the following set of instructions:

    1. Make 1% solution of apple juice in alcohol.

                Producing Effective SOPs

2. Measure the pH.

3. Make a 1:10 dilution of the existing diluted solution.

4. Measure the pH again.

5. Until you have 10 pH readings, go to step 3.

6. Examine the data for linearity.

Identify the problems with these instructions.

4 Your manager has told you, after a request from QA, to improve an SOP. The process described in this SOP requires a calculation and most of the users are either making wrong calculations or their results are inconsistent with each other. How will you improve the next version of this SOP?

5 Describe how the *Plan-Do-Check-Act* quality cycle can be applied to the whole SOP system in a company.

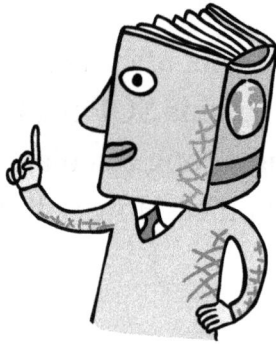

Producing Effective SOPs

4

Living With Approved SOPs

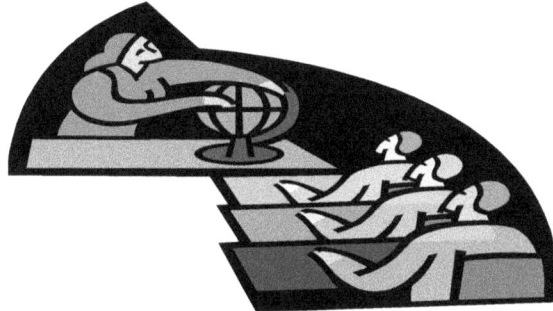

1. Big Picture

2. SOP Training

3. Following an SOP

4. Data Entry and Comments

5. Monitoring and Controlling SOPs

6. Changing SOPs

7. Destroying SOPs

8. Summary and Conclusions

9. Self Test Exercises

Living with Approved SOPs: Big Picture

You are required by law to comply with the approved SOPs. Living with an approved SOP includes:

- Training the SOP users
- Following the SOP
- Monitoring and controlling the SOP
- Writing data and comments into a lab book or a log book while following the SOP, for example, performing a procedure according to the SOP
- Suggesting changes to the SOP
- Suggesting a new SOP
- Implementing changes, that is, modifying an approved SOP
- Getting approval for the modified SOP
- Making an existing SOP obsolete
- Destroying an existing SOP

Training the SOP Users

- Assess the SOP training needs:
  - Perform cost benefit analysis.
  - Remember, the cost of correcting errors caught by inspection is much higher than preventing the error.
  - Consider that the training can help in preventing the errors.
- Determine training requirements:
  - What will be included in the training?
  - Who will be included in the training?
  - What results do you need from the training?
- Based on the needs, requirements, and the situation, the training can be one or more of the following types:
  - One on one
  - Classroom
  - Online
  - On the job
- Training needs may arise from:
  - New SOPs have been written
  - Newly hired employees need to follow the SOP system
  - One or more current employees making too many mistakes in following the SOPs

Living with Approved SOPs

Following SOPs

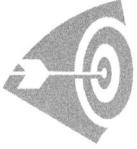

Following an SOP means performing the tasks about which the SOP is written according to the SOP.

Some Tips:

- Read the SOP carefully and re-read the SOP often.

- Keep a copy of the SOP easily accessible while you work.

- Make sure you understand each step before executing it. Check your understanding.

- If you cannot follow the step for whatever reason, do not execute the step. Stop and communicate with the appropriate person.

- Following SOP is not the place and time for innovation.

While you are performing a procedure (task) according to the SOP, you will often be recording some data in a notebook such as a lab book or a log book

Recording Data

Find out if your company has an SOP about recording data or making comments. Here are some generally acceptable rules or guidelines:

Data Entry:

- Record the data in a designated notebook.

- Sign the data entry with date.

- If you need to cancel a record, cross it with a single line, put your initial with date.

- Use the ball point pen or ink pen as opposed to lead pencil so that it could not be easily erased.

- Be honest in recording the data, do not make it up or modify it. If you do not believe the data, or if you think there is something wrong that might have produced the wrong results, you can write your comment, but do not make up (or modify) the data.

Writing Comments

- It may include comments about the procedure, data, and the SOP.

- Be precise and professional in making your comments.

- You may add comments to help other users.

- Add comments for an unusual observation such as about the data or about the SOP.

- Write a comment about a deviation, for example, you made a mistake that produced wrong data.

- Write necessary comments about the data such as:

  o Wrong entry was made accidentally

  o Data was entered late

  o There was an error in the calculation

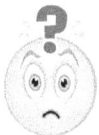

How do I write comments?

Writing Comments: Dos and Don'ts

Dos:

- Record a deviation, e.g., a mistake you made
- Notes to clarify something
- Rewrite if the handwriting of the first write was bad
- Record an anomaly or unusual observation
- Be professional

Don'ts:

- Opinions as opposed to facts
- Emotions
- Comments undermining other's work or the SOP, or admission of guilt:
  - Example: *This is all an artifact.*

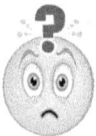

What if somebody want to make a change in the SOP?

Living with Approved SOPs

Monitoring and Controlling SOPs

Monitoring and controlling SOPs include:

- Making sure the SOPs are being followed
- Monitoring the effectiveness of SOPs that are being followed
- Putting in place the change control system that facilitates:
    - Making a change request
    - Evaluating the change request
    - Approving or disapproving the change request
    - Implementing the approved changes

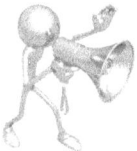

Your company must have a change control system in place, and only the changes approved through this system should be implemented.

Keeping the Change History

It's crucial to keep the change history:

- Document the change properly that includes:
    - When was the change made and why?
    - Who approved it?
- Link the change history to the document so that it can be easily traced when needed.

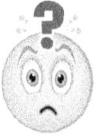

What does change to an SOP include?

Living with Approved SOPs

Changing an SOP

Change to an SOP includes:

- **Modifying an SOP**

- **Making an SOP obsolete**

- **Archiving an SOP**

- **Destroying an SOP.** Yes, copies of the outdated or superceded SOPs can be destroyed according to an approved procedure.

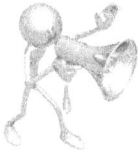

Destroying a document is a serious activity. The committee that would approve destroying an SOP must consist of at least two individuals. Your company may also have an SOP about destroying SOPs or other documents.

Following SOPs in the Light of GMPs

- Follow your SOP accurately and exactly.

- Double check the critical steps if needed (for example if you are new). have a colleague check critical steps.

- Record the data carefully and honestly.

- Check for anomalies, errors, and gaps.

- Report troubles and unusual observations to the management.

- Be professional in writing comments.

Summary and Conclusions

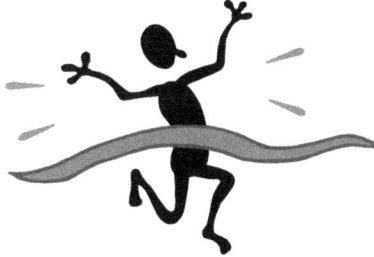

- The tasks after an SOP is approved include needed training, following the SOP, monitoring the effectiveness of the SOP, and controlling the changes to the SOP.

- An approved SOP must be followed; this is the law.

- Changes to an SOP must be approved through proper procedure before they are implemented.

- An SOP must only be destroyed according to an approved procedure or SOP.

- Data must be recorded accurately and honestly.

- Be professional in writing comments.

Self Test Exercises

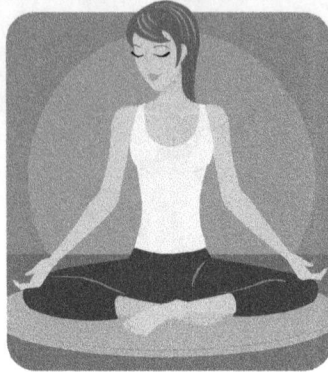

1 What's wrong with the following comments that a research assistant made in the lab book?

1. *This assay never works.*

2. *I think I have collected enough data and built some confidence. Therefore, I have extrapolated/guessed a couple of last data points required by the SOP: I gotta run...*

3. *This SOP stinks*

2 You are a research associate working in your lab. You are in the middle of performing a procedure according to an SOP. You have run into a step in the SOP that cannot be executed the way it is written. You are an expert in the field and you know what you are doing. Which of the following is the correct course of action?

A. You are an expert and you know what you are doing; so ignore the step in the SOP and execute the step as you think is correct.

B. Stop performing the procedure and take the issue to your manager.

C. Make a correction to the SOP and continue performing the procedure.

D. Perform the step the way you think is correct, and report the error in the SOP to the QA department.

3 Which of the following is true about destroying an SOP or making it obsolete?

A. The SOP can be destroyed by the author of the SOP.

B. The SOP can be destroyed by the users of the SOP if there is a unanimous consent among the users.

C. The procedure for destroying an SOP should include the consent of at least two individuals.

D. It's illegal to destroy any approved SOP.

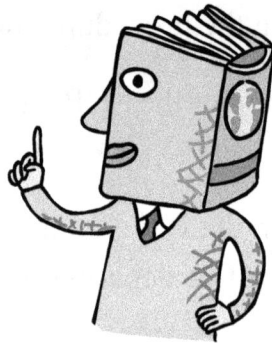

Living with Approved SOPs

5

Process Based Approach to SOPS

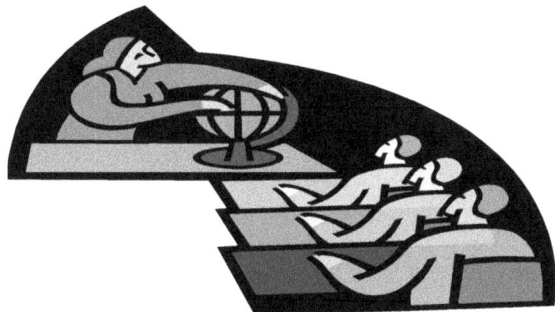

1. Process Based Approach: Definition

2. What is a process?

3. Following an SOP

4. Data Entry and Comments

5. Monitoring and Controlling SOPs

6. Destroying SOPs

7. Summary and Conclusions

8. Self Test Exercises

Process Based Approach to SOPS

Introducing the Process Based Approach to SOPs

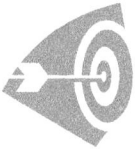

The process based SOP approach is the approach that is used to perform SOP related tasks in terms of processes.

Examples of SOP Related Tasks:

- Writing an SOP
- Reviewing an SOP
- Approving an SOP
- Following an SOP
- Monitoring SOP, for example, monitoring its performance and effectiveness
- Controlling SOP, for example, controlling the changes to the SOP

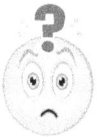

By the way, what is a process?

What is a Process?

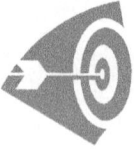

A process is a set of related actions directed to produce an output.

Example: Think of making coffee, or developing a schedule for your project.

Each process consists of three elements described in the following:

♦   **Input.** Consists of the raw data that is needed to start the process. For example, the list of activities that need to be scheduled is one of several input items to the process that will be used to develop the schedule of a project.

♦   **Tools and Techniques.** The tools and methods that are used to operate on the input to produce output. For example, project management software that helps to develop a schedule is a tool used in the schedule development process.

♦   **Output**. The outcome or the result of a process. Each process contains at least one output item; otherwise there is no point in performing the process. For example an output item of the schedule development process is, well, the project schedule.

Three Main Steps in Any Process

1. Gather input
2. Operate on the input by using tools and techniques to produce output
3. Collect the output

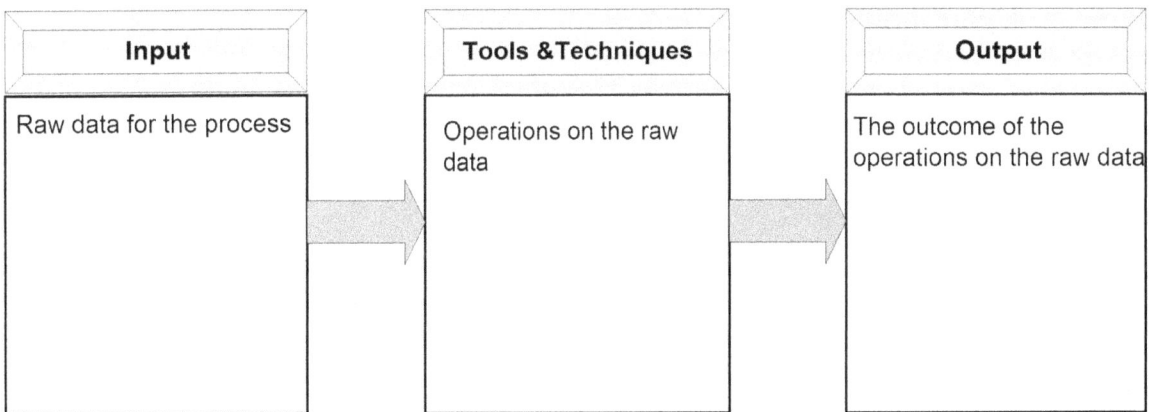

Input	Tools &Techniques	Output
Raw data for the process	Operations on the raw data	The outcome of the operations on the raw data

Three elements of a process: input, tools & techniques, and output

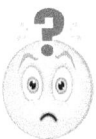

Can you please give some examples of SOP related processes?

Examples of SOP Processes

- Write SOPs
- Review SOPs
- Approve SOPs
- Follow SOPs
- Monitor SOPs
- Control SOPs

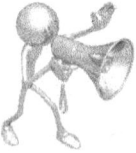

On the next pages, these SOP processes are presented in terms of their input, tools and techniques, and output. The lists of input, tools and techniques, and output are in no way complete. These examples are presented here just to illustrate the process based approach. In context of your SOP, organization, and industry, you can make your own lists of input, tools and techniques, and output. You can also design new SOP related processes as needed.

Process Based Approach to SOPS

The Write SOP Process

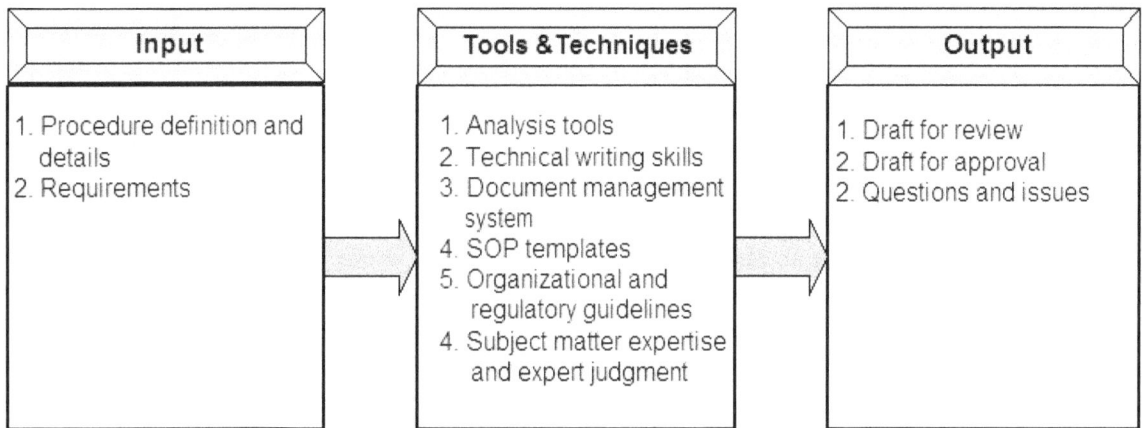

Input	Tools & Techniques	Output
1. Procedure definition and details 2. Requirements	1. Analysis tools 2. Technical writing skills 3. Document management system 4. SOP templates 5. Organizational and regulatory guidelines 4. Subject matter expertise and expert judgment	1. Draft for review 2. Draft for approval 2. Questions and issues

The write SOP process

The Review SOP Process

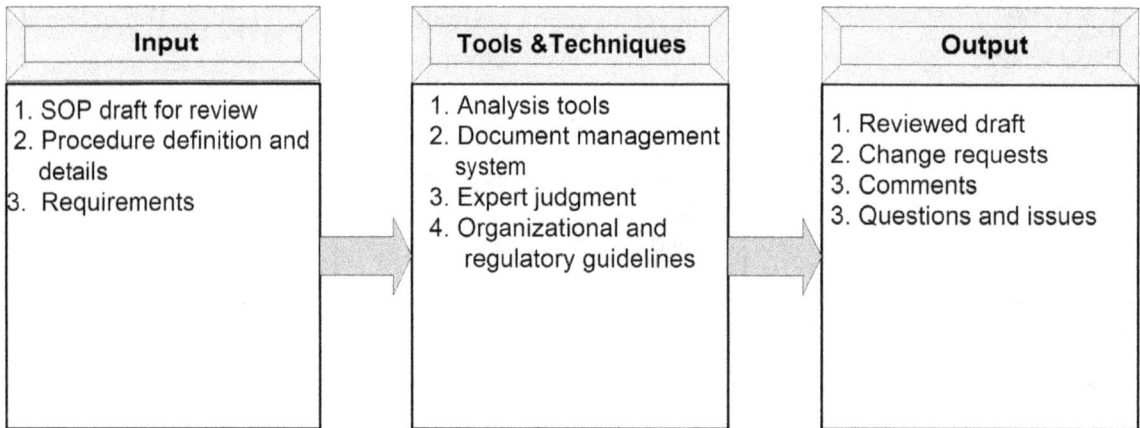

Input	Tools &Techniques	Output
1. SOP draft for review 2. Procedure definition and details 3. Requirements	1. Analysis tools 2. Document management system 3. Expert judgment 4. Organizational and regulatory guidelines	1. Reviewed draft 2. Change requests 3. Comments 3. Questions and issues

The review sop process

The Approve SOP Process

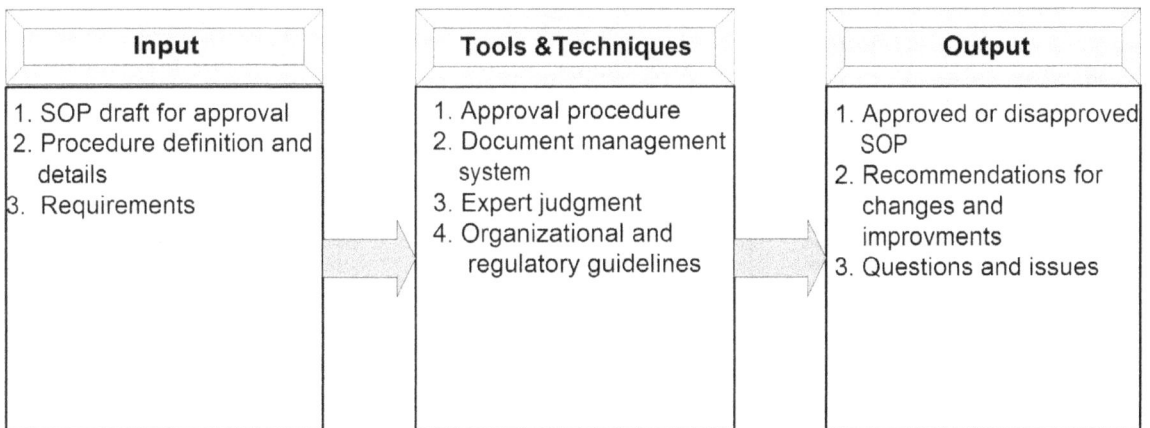

Input	Tools &Techniques	Output

1. SOP draft for approval
2. Procedure definition and
   details
3. Requirements
	1. Approval procedure
	2. Document management
	   system
	3. Expert judgment
	4. Organizational and
	   regulatory guidelines
		1. Approved or disapproved
		   SOP
		2. Recommendations for
		   changes and
		   improvments
		3. Questions and issues

The approve sop process

The Follow SOP Process

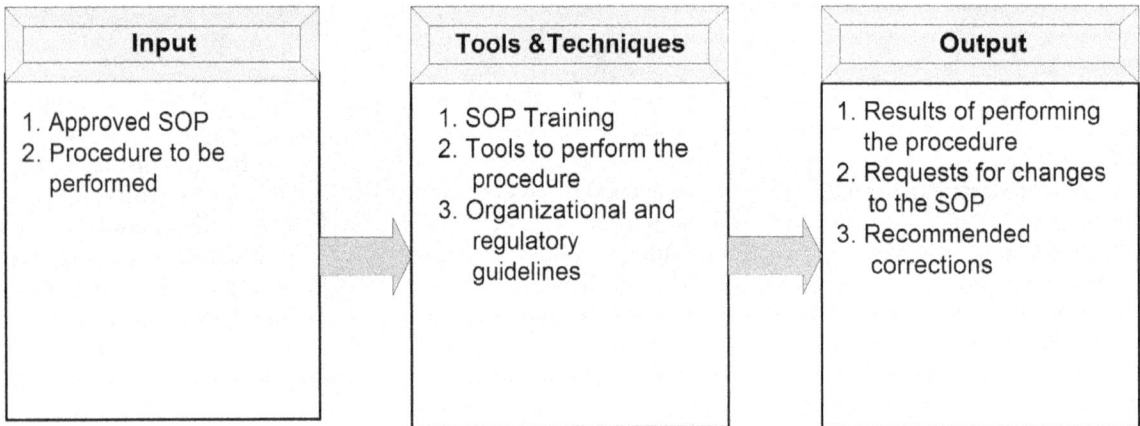

Input	Tools &Techniques	Output
1. Approved SOP 2. Procedure to be performed	1. SOP Training 2. Tools to perform the procedure 3. Organizational and regulatory guidelines	1. Results of performing the procedure 2. Requests for changes to the SOP 3. Recommended corrections

The follow sop process

Process Based Approach to SOPS

The Monitor SOP Process

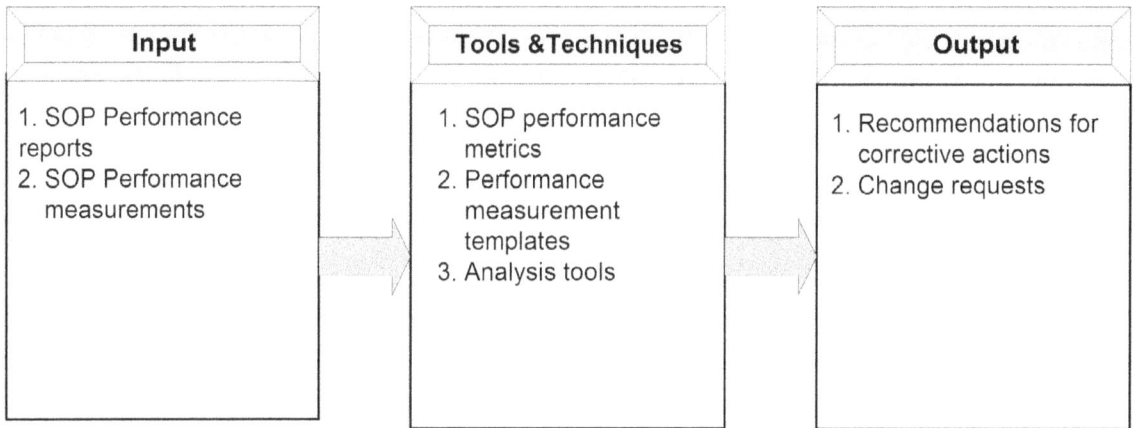

Input	Tools &Techniques	Output
1. SOP Performance reports 2. SOP Performance measurements	1. SOP performance metrics 2. Performance measurement templates 3. Analysis tools	1. Recommendations for corrective actions 2. Change requests

The monitor sop process

The Control SOP Process

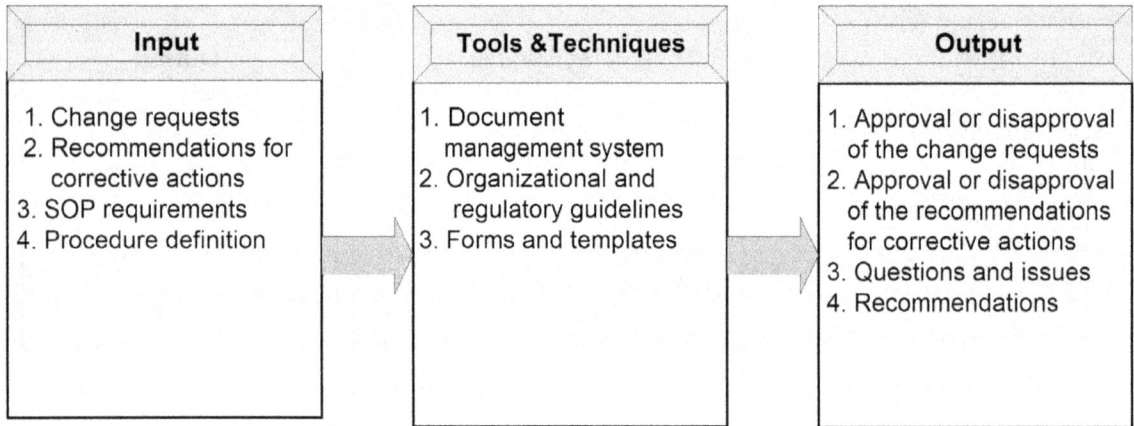

Input	Tools &Techniques	Output
1. Change requests 2. Recommendations for corrective actions 3. SOP requirements 4. Procedure definition	1. Document management system 2. Organizational and regulatory guidelines 3. Forms and templates	1. Approval or disapproval of the change requests 2. Approval or disapproval of the recommendations for corrective actions 3. Questions and issues 4. Recommendations

The control sop process

Benefits of the Process Based Approach to SOPs

- Enforces planning before execution, which improves:
  - quality
  - performance
  - efficiency
- Minimizes the possibility of gaps or surprises.
- Minimizes risk
- Facilitates doing the right thing and avoiding or catching errors and mistakes.

Summary and Conclusions

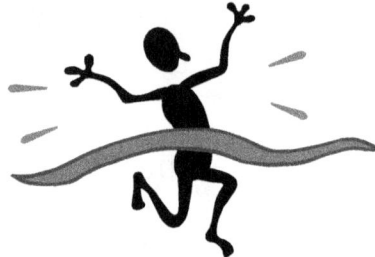

- The process based SOP approach is the approach that is used to perform SOP related tasks in terms of processes.

- A process is a set of related actions directed to produce an output.

- A process has three main elements: input, tools and techniques, and output.

- Related SOP tasks (or actions) can be grouped into a process.

- SOP related tasks can be grouped into several processes. Following are some examples:

  - Write SOP
  - Review SOP
  - Approve SOP
  - Monitor SOP

- o   Control SOP

- The process based approach to SOP enforces planning, which helps generate the following benefits:

  - o   Improvement in efficiency, performance, and quality.

  - o   Minimization of risk, and the probability of gaps, errors, and mistakes

Self Test Exercises

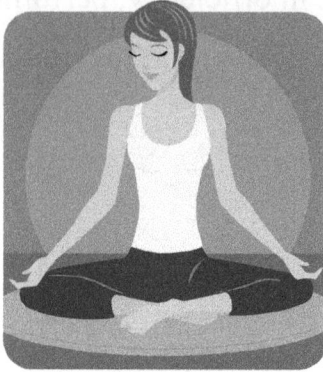

1 What are the three main elements of a process?

2 Give an example of a process in which the SOP templates will be an output.

3 You are designing a process: destroy SOP. List some input items to this process.

4 You are designing a process: destroy SOP. List some tools and techniques for this process.

5 The traditional way of making Indian tea is the following:

1. Put some tea leaves and sugar in the water.

2. Boil this mixture of tea leaves, sugar, and water.

3. After a few minutes of boiling, put some milk into the mixture.

4. Give it a couple of more boils.

5. Take the pot off the stove.

6. The tea is ready to be served.

What are the input, tools and techniques, and output of the make Indian tea process?

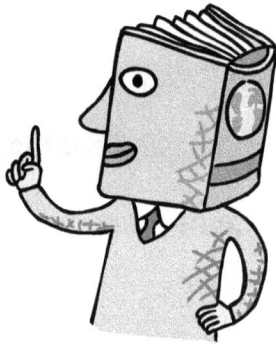

Process Based Approach to SOPS

Solutions to Self Test Exercises

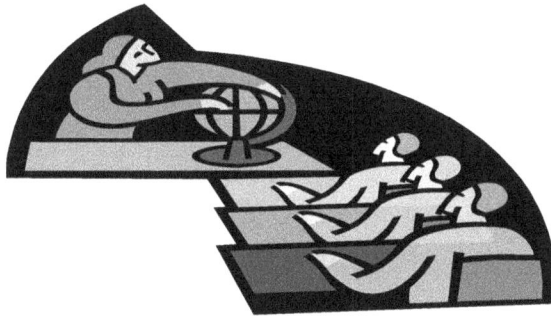

Solutions

Module 1

1. What is an SOP?

Solution:

Standard Operating Procedure.

Detailed, written instructions to achieve uniformity and consistency in performing a specific process or procedure.

2. True or False: SOPs in clinical industry are documents standardized for the whole industry, which describe how to perform certain operations.

Solution:

False.

SOPs are not industry standards, and are usually written at an organizational level.

3. True or False: SOPs are only used in biotechnology and health industry.

Solution:

False.

SOPs can be used in any number of industries to achieve the benefits they offer.

4. True or False. SOPs are only used to meet regulatory requirements.

Solution:

False.

To meet regulatory requirements is one of many advantages of SOPs.

5. Each SOP has a start point of an operation and the finish point. In SOP 1.1 for cooking pizza presented in module 1, identify the start point and the finish point.

Solution:

Start point. We are in the kitchen with an oven and uncooked pizza.

Finish point. The cooked pizza has been taken out of the oven.

Another SOP, e.g. how to serve pizza, may start from where this SOP ends.

6. SOPs often have assumptions, for example, they may assume that there is something that the user already knows and does not need to be written down. Identify at least one assumption in SOP 1.1 for cooking pizza.

Solution:

Users already know how to safely take pizza out of the hot oven.

7. An SOP may have a flexibility built into it. Identify at least one flexibility built into SOP 1.1 for cooking pizza.

Solution:

Steps 5 to 7 represent flexibility of how well done you want your pizza.

Solutions to Self Test Exercises

Solutions

Module 2

1. You have just made an SOP obsolete. There are three existing SOPs that refer to this SOP. What will you do to maintain the effectiveness of those SOPs?

Solution:

Make sure those SOPs (or any other SOP) do not refer to this SOP that has been made obsolete. Either remove those references by putting the required additional information into those SOPs or replace those references with references to appropriate existing SOPs.

2. Most employees have deviated step 5 of your SOP most of the time. What is the most likely problem? Suggest a solution.

Solution:

Because most of the people are deviating on step 5, most likely the problem is with the step 5. For example, there may be an error in step 5, it may not be well written, or it may be impractical to follow.

The solution depends on the problem. For example if the problem is with the clarity of step 5, the solution is to re-write it clearly.

3. One employee has deviated step 5 of your SOP most of the times. Other employees are using this SOP as well, and they are not deviating. What is the most likely problem? Suggest a solution.

Solution:

Because only one person is deviating on step 5, most likely problem is that for some reason that person is unable to follow step 5. An appropriate individual should communicate with that person, find out the reason about the deviation, and fix the problem. The solution may involve training.

4. Changes in SOPs must be controlled by:

    A. Authors of the SOPs

    B. QA

    C. CEO of the company

    D. Manager of the users

Solution:

B

Solutions

Module 3

1. You see a signboard that reads the following:

Chemicals that are known to be dangerous to your health are used in this facility!

This warning is suffering from which pitfall?

Solution:

Lack of specificity:

1. What specifically are those chemicals?

2. How exactly are those chemicals dangerous?

3. Those chemicals are dangerous according to whom?

2. What are the possible results of vague instructions for a procedure?

Solution:

1. Inconsistent execution by different users.

2. Wrong execution with possibly fatal results.

3. Read the following set of instructions:

1. Make 1% solution of apple juice in alcohol.

2. Measure the pH.

3. Make a 1:10 dilution of the existing diluted solution.

4. Measure the pH again.

5. Until you have 10 pH readings, go to step 3.

6. Examine the data for linearity.

What are the problems with these instructions?

Answer:

1. 1% solution of apple juice: is this percentage by weight or by volume?

2. Measure the pH with what device? If you don't mention, different users will measure pH by using different devices and therefore will get readings with different accuracies.

3. 1: 10 dilution in what? Water? Alcohol? Again, because solvent is not specified, different users will use different solvents and will get different results.

4. Examine the data for linearity. Which data and linearity against what?

4. Your manager has told you, after a request from QA, to improve an SOP. The process described in this SOP requires a calculation and most of the users are either making wrong calculations or their results are inconsistent with each other. How will you improve the next version of this SOP?

Solution:

One or more of the following steps can be taken to improve the SOP:

1. Make the instructions about the calculation very clear such as number of significant figures needed.

2. Give an example of this calculation.

5. Describe how the *Plan-Do-Check-Act* quality cycle can be applied to the whole SOP system in a company.

Solution:

The Quality Cycle Stage	Corresponding SOP System Activity
Plan	Plan for implementing the SOP system, for example, what SOPs you need, what re the requirements, who will approve them, etc.
Do	Write, review, and approve SOPs
Check	Monitor and control the SOPs. Make sure they are being followed. Suggest changes to existing SOPs or suggest new SOPs if required for improvement.
Act	Implement the changes.

Solutions

Module 4

1. What's wrong with the following comments that a research assistant made in the lab book?

1. *This assay never works.*

2. *I think I have collected enough data and built some confidence. Therefore, I have extrapolated/guessed a couple of last data points required by the SOP: I gotta run...*

3. *This SOP stinks*

Solution:

1 and 3. Not specific and not professional.

2. Admission of guilt; liability risk. You must not be making up data in the first place.

2. You are a research associate and working in your lab. You are in the middle of performing a procedure according to an SOP. You have run into a step in the SOP that cannot be executed the way it is written. You are an expert in the field and you know what you are doing. Which of the following is the correct course of action?

A. You are an expert and you know what you are doing; so ignore the step in the SOP and execute the step as you think is correct.

B. Stop performing the procedure and take the issue to your manager.

C. Make a correction to the SOP and continue performing the procedure.

D. Perform the step the way you think is correct, and report the error in the SOP to the QA department.

Solution:

B is the correct answer.

3. Which of the following is true about destroying an SOP or making it obsolete?

A. The SOP can be destroyed by the author of the SOP.

B. The SOP can be destroyed by the users of the SOP if there is a unanimous consent among the users.

C. The procedure for destroying an SOP should include the consent of at least two individuals.

D. It's illegal to destroy any approved SOP.

Solution:

C is the correct answer.

Solutions

Module 5

1. What are the three main elements of a process?

Solution:

1. Input

2. Tools and techniques

3. Output

2. Give an example of a process in which SOP templates will be an output.

Solution:

Think of a process of planning an SOP system for your company. In this process SOP templates will be one of the output items.

3. You are designing a process: destroy SOP. List some input items to this process.

Solution:

1. The SOP to be destroyed

2. Approval for destroying the SOP

4. You are designing a process: destroy SOP. List some tools and techniques for this process.

Solution:

1. Paper shredding tool

2. Organizational and regulatory guidelines

5. The traditional way of making Indian tea is the following:

1. Put some tea leaves and sugar in the water.

2. Boil this mixture of tea leaves, sugar, and water.

3. After a few minutes of boiling, put some milk into the mixture.

4. Give it a couple of more boils.

5. Take the pot off the stove.

6. The tea is ready to be served.

What are the input, tools and techniques, and output of the *make Indian tea* process?

Solution:

Input	Tools &Techniques	Output
1. Water 2. Tea leaves 3. Sugar 4. Milk	1. Stove or some other tool to generate heat energy. 2. Tea pot	1. Indian tea 2. Waste such as used tea leves

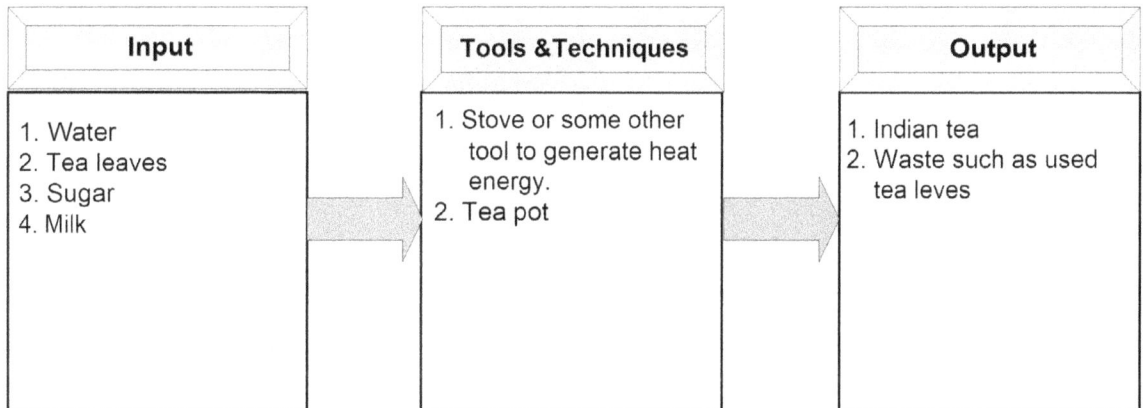

The make Indian tea process: input, tools & techniques, and output

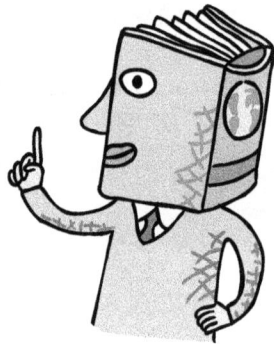

Solutions to Self Test Exercises

Some example SOP Templates

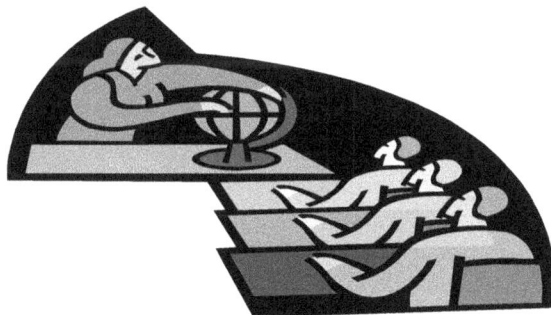

SOP #   Author:_____

Title: Performing The Gram Stain Procedures in the Research Lab

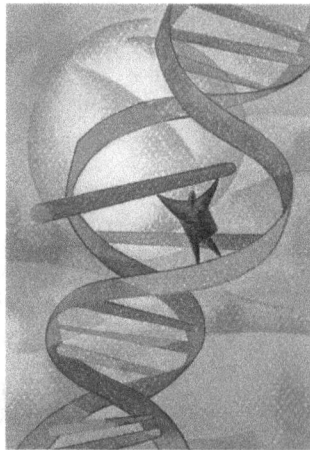

Table of Contents

The Gram Staining Procedure: An Example SOP Template

3. Apparatus and materials

4. Background Information

5. Procedures

6. References

7. Change History

Purpose

State the purpose of this SOP, for example:

To perform the gram stain procedure in order to differentiate between gram negative organisms and gram positive organisms.

Scope

To whom this SOP applies and to whom it does not

Apparatus and Materials

List the apparatus used in the procedure such as:

- Bunsen burner
- Microscope
- Microscope slides
- Distilled water

List the material such as reagents:

- Crystal violet
- Iodine solution
- Ethanol (decolorizer)
- Safranin (the counterstainer)

Background Information

Explain the scientific background and theory behind gram staining and how it works.

Procedures

List the steps for the procedures involved in this task such as preparing the bacteria slide, staining, examining under the microscope, and recording observations.

References

List of references for the information in this document

Change History

List of changes (with dates and reasons) made to this document

Approval

Approved by:

Name_____

Signature_____

Date_____

The Gram Staining Procedure: An Example SOP Template

Cleaning in the R&D Lab

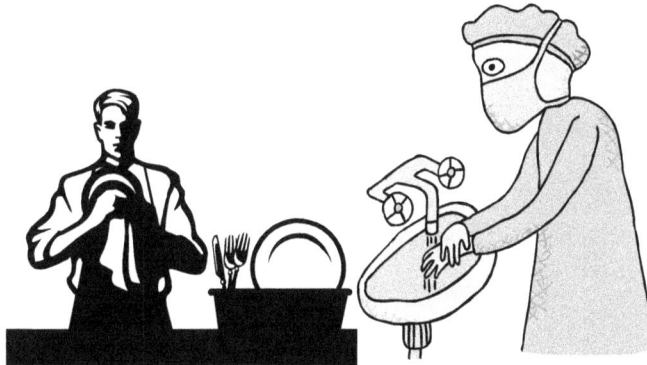

Table of Contents

5. Procedures

6. General Notes

7. Change History

Cleaning in the R&D Lab: An Example SOP Template

Purpose

State the purpose of this SOP, for example:

General instructions on cleaning surfaces and small reusable objects in the research and development laboratory

Scope

To whom this SOP applies and to whom it does not

The objects (to be cleaned) to which this SOP applies

Materials

List the material used such as:

- Sanisol
- Detergent
- Deionized
- Distilled water
- Tap water

Background Information

Provide and explain necessary background information such as difference between deionized water and distilled water, cleaning and sterilizing, and soaking and scrubbing.

Procedures

List the steps for the procedures involved such as cleaning surfaces, cleaning glassware, and drying.

General Notes

Any useful information not covered in the background section such as choices for different kinds of detergents.

Change History

List of changes (with dates and reasons) made to this document

Approval

Approved by:

Name_____

Signature_____

Date_____

SOP #   Author:_____

Laboratory Safety Manual

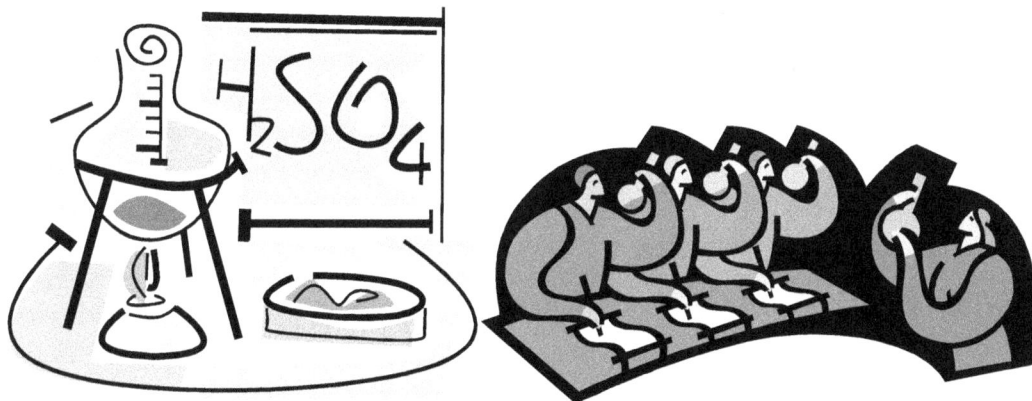

Table of Contents

4. Responsibility Assignments

5. Laboratory Equipment

6. Laboratory Safety Guidelines

7. Chemical Handling and Processing

8. Laboratory Closeouts

9. Appendices

10. Change History

The Laboratory Safety Manual: An Example SOP Template

Purpose

State the purpose of this SOP, for example:

To help the staff carry out research programs in a safe and healthy lab environment.

Scope

To whom this SOP applies and to whom it does not

The objects (to be cleaned) to which this SOP applies

Emergency Telephone Numbers

List of telephone numbers for different emergency events such as fire, chemical spill, radiation accident, biological accident, and indoor air quality concerns

Responsibility Assignments

Description of safety related responsibility assignments such as the individual lab staff members are responsible for their own safety and the laboratory manager is responsible for controlling hazards in the laboratory.

Laboratory Equipment

List the laboratory equipment and the safety related information about the equipment.

Laboratory Safety Guidelines

State safety guidelines about different aspects of the lab such as hazards, clothing and footwear, food and drink, spills and cleanup, electrical safety, visitors, first aid, and so on.

Safety Procedures

List the steps for different safety related procedures, for example, what to do in an event of fire. Here you can also refer to other SOPs.

Laboratory Closeouts

Describe the proper procedure to close the lab at the end of the day, for the weekend, and for holidays, for example, what needs to be done before closure and who needs to be informed.

Change History

List of changes (with dates and reasons) made to this document

Approval

Approved by:

Name_____

Signature_____

Date_____

Glossary

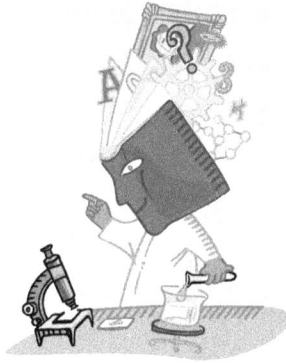

cGMP. The current Good Manufacturing Practices enforced by FDA. The World Health Organization and the European Union have their own versions of GMP.

Change control system (CCS). A collection of formal documented procedures that specifies how certain entities such as project plans and scopes, and other documents will be controlled, changed, and approved.

Configuration management system (CMS). A system that manages the following characteristics of a product: identity, consistency, change control, status accounting, verification, and auditing.

Content management system (CMS). A content management system (CMS). A computerized system used to create, store, edit, control, and retrieve (or publish) content in a consistent and automated fashion.

Document management system (DMS). A computerized system that consists of computers and software programs to manage documents.

FDA. The U.S. Food and Drug Administration. An agency of the United States Department of Health and Human Services that is responsible for the safety regulation of most types of dietary supplements, drugs and other health and medical related products, cosmetics, and medical devices.

GCP. Good Clinical Practices; an international quality standard of ICH, an international body that defines standards, which governments can transpose into regulations for clinical trials involving human subjects.

GMP. Good manufacturing practice; a requirement for manufacturers of foods and medications including biotechnology products, pharmaceuticals, and active pharmaceutical ingredients in order to ensure the required quality of medications and related products.

ICH. The International Conference on Harmonization of Technical Requirements for Registration of Pharmaceuticals for Human Use; a project or platform that brings together the regulatory authorities of Europe, Japan and the United States along with the experts from the pharmaceutical industry in the three regions to discuss scientific and technical aspects of pharmaceutical product registration.

IRB. Institutional review board; a formal committee that has been designated to approve, monitor, and review biomedical and behavioral research involving humans with the aim to protect the rights and welfare of the research (or study) subjects. IRBs may be formed under different names such as ethical review board (IRB) or independent ethics committee (IEC).

Metrics. A system used to evaluate an entity such as a process, document, or performance quantitatively. It specifies a set of parameters that will be measured, a procedure to measure them, and a way to interpret the measurements.

Process. A set of related actions directed to produce an output. A process has input that produces output when acted upon by using some tools and techniques.

Process Based SOP Approach. The approach that is used to perform SOP related tasks in terms of processes; introduced by Paul Sanghera in 2008.

Quality. The degree to which the characteristics of a product meet the planned requirements and objectives.

QA. Quality assurance; a system that includes activities and processes designed to ensure that the development and maintenance processes in place are good enough to ensure the final product will meet the planned objectives.

QC. Quality control; a system that consists of activities and processes to control the quality, for example, to evaluate the product to verify if it meets the required quality and to provide a review. Usually companies have one department that includes quality assurance and quality control.

SOP. Standard operating procedure; a document that contains accurate and detailed instructions to perform a process, procedure, or operation.

Your Notes

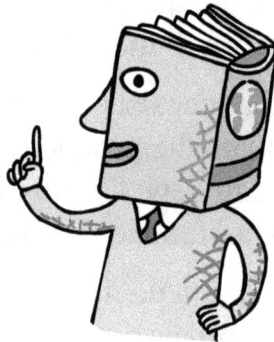

Your Notes

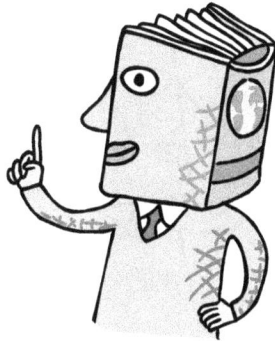

Your Notes

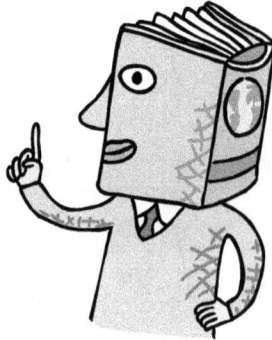

SOP Workshop: Glossary

Your Notes

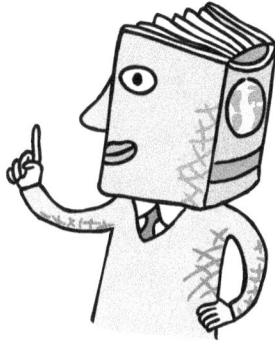

The End

www.ingramcontent.com/pod-product-compliance
Lightning Source LLC
Chambersburg PA
CBHW080556220326
41599CB00032B/6503